SOMATIC EXERCISE

FOR BEGINNERS

A Comprehensive Guide To Enhance Flexibility, Relieve Pain, Reduce Stress, And Improve Mind-Body Connection

ROBERT LUGO

INTRODUCTION

Somatic exercises offer a unique approach to physical wellness, focusing on the mind-body connection and enhancing body awareness.

These exercises encompass a range of movements and techniques designed to improve flexibility, posture, and overall well-being. For beginners, somatic exercises provide an accessible entry point into holistic health practices, offering benefits that extend beyond the physical realm.

One of the key concepts in somatic exercises is the emphasis on awareness. Unlike traditional fitness routines that often prioritize external results, such as muscle growth or weight loss, somatic exercises encourage individuals to tune into their internal sensations. This heightened awareness allows beginners to identify areas of tension, imbalance, or restricted movement within their bodies.

By honing in on these areas, individuals can then work towards releasing tension, improving mobility, and restoring natural movement patterns.

Another fundamental aspect of somatic exercises is the focus on gentle, mindful movements. Rather than pushing the body to its limits or engaging in high-intensity workouts, somatic exercises advocate for slow, controlled movements that promote relaxation and ease. This approach is especially beneficial for beginners who may be new to physical activity or have limited mobility.

By starting with gentle movements, individuals can gradually build strength, flexibility, and coordination without the risk of strain or injury.

Furthermore, somatic exercises often incorporate principles of breath awareness and relaxation. Learning to synchronize breath with movement not only enhances the efficacy of the exercises but also cultivates a sense of calm and presence. For beginners, this integration of breathwork can be particularly beneficial in reducing stress, improving mental clarity, and fostering a deeper connection between mind and body.

The benefits of somatic exercises for beginners are manifold. One of the primary advantages is the promotion of better posture and alignment.

Many individuals, especially in today's sedentary lifestyle, struggle with poor posture due to prolonged sitting or improper movement patterns.

Somatic exercises help beginners re-educate their bodies, encouraging proper alignment of the spine, shoulders, and hips. This, in turn, can alleviate common issues like back pain, neck tension, and postural imbalances.

Additionally, somatic exercises can enhance flexibility and mobility, making everyday movements easier and more fluid. By targeting specific muscle groups and releasing tension, beginners can experience an increased range of motion and freedom in their movements.

This is particularly beneficial for older adults or individuals recovering from injuries, as improved flexibility can enhance independence and quality of life.

Another notable benefit of somatic exercises is stress reduction and relaxation. The mindful approach to movement, coupled with breath awareness techniques, helps beginners unwind and release built-up tension.

This can have profound effects on overall well-being, promoting better sleep, mood regulation, and resilience to stressors.

Moreover, somatic exercises can be adapted to suit individual needs and abilities, making them highly inclusive and accessible. Beginners of all ages and fitness levels can participate in somatic practices, tailoring the exercises to their unique goals and limitations.

This adaptability not only ensures safety but also encourages a sense of empowerment and autonomy in one's wellness journey.

This manual serves as a comprehensive guide for beginners embarking on their somatic exercise journey. It provides detailed explanations of various somatic techniques, accompanied by step-by-step instructions and illustrations to facilitate learning.

Each chapter delves into different aspects of somatic exercises, from foundational movements to advanced practices, offering a progressive approach to skill development.

Furthermore, this manual addresses common challenges and misconceptions that beginners may encounter, providing practical tips and troubleshooting strategies. By demystifying somatic exercises and offering clear guidance, this manual empowers beginners to confidently explore and integrate somatic practices into their daily lives.

In essence, this manual is a valuable resource for beginners seeking to enhance their physical and mental well-being through somatic exercises.

By embracing the principles of awareness, gentle movement, and breathwork, individuals can unlock the transformative potential of somatic practices and embark on a journey of self-discovery and holistic wellness.

CHAPTER 1
Understanding Somatics

In somatic exercises for beginners, understanding the core principles is crucial for a comprehensive grasp of this holistic approach to movement and well-being. Somatics emphasizes the mind-body connection, focusing on awareness, sensation, and the integration of these elements for improved function and health. This exploration delves into the principles of somatic exercises, the intricate relationship between the mind and body, and the pivotal role of awareness and sensation in somatic practices.

The principles of somatic exercises revolve around the concept of sensory-motor learning, where movement is not just a mechanical action but a deeply integrated process involving the brain, muscles, and sensory feedback. Central to somatics is the idea that habitual movement patterns, often developed in response to stress, injury, or environmental factors, can lead to chronic tension, pain, and restricted mobility. Through somatic exercises, individuals can reeducate their nervous system, release tension, and restore balanced movement patterns.

One key principle of somatic exercises is the focus on internal sensing or interoception. Interoception refers to the ability to sense and perceive internal bodily states, such as muscle tension, breathing patterns, and emotional responses. By developing greater interoceptive awareness, individuals can become more attuned to subtle changes within their bodies, allowing for a deeper understanding of how stress, emotions, and movement patterns interact.

Another fundamental principle is the concept of pandiculation, a term coined by Thomas Hanna, the founder of Clinical Somatic Education. Pandiculation involves a voluntary contraction of muscles followed by a slow, controlled release. This action engages the sensory-motor loop, resetting muscle length and promoting relaxation. Through pandiculation, individuals can release chronic muscular contraction, improve muscle function, and reduce pain.

Furthermore, somatic exercises emphasize the importance of slow, mindful movement. Unlike traditional exercise approaches that often focus on external cues or forceful exertion, somatics encourage gentle, exploratory movements guided by internal sensation.

This approach fosters a sense of agency and self-discovery, allowing individuals to develop a deeper connection with their bodies and cultivate greater body awareness.

The mind-body connection lies at the heart of somatic practices. Somatic exercises recognize that mental and emotional states can profoundly influence physical well-being. Stress, anxiety, and unresolved emotions can manifest as muscular tension and movement restrictions. Through somatic awareness techniques such as breathwork, mindfulness, and imagery, individuals can address these psychosomatic patterns, promoting relaxation, emotional resilience, and overall vitality.

In somatic exercises, the role of awareness and sensation is paramount. Awareness refers to the conscious attention directed toward internal bodily experiences, movement quality, and sensory feedback. By cultivating mindful awareness during movement practices, individuals can identify areas of tension, track changes in muscle tone, and refine movement patterns. This heightened awareness fosters self-regulation and empowers individuals to make conscious choices that support optimal movement and well-being.

Sensation, on the other hand, encompasses the felt experience of movement, including proprioception (awareness of body position in space), kinesthesia (perception of movement), and tactile sensations. Somatic exercises encourage individuals to explore subtle sensations during movement, such as the lengthening of muscles, the coordination of breath and movement, and the integration of whole-body alignment. Through focused attention on sensation, individuals can refine movement quality, improve motor control, and enhance overall movement efficiency.

Moreover, somatic exercises emphasize the role of relaxation and release in optimizing movement function. Chronic stress and muscular tension can disrupt neuromuscular coordination, leading to inefficient movement patterns and discomfort.

By incorporating techniques such as progressive relaxation, breath awareness, and gentle stretching, somatic exercises promote a state of relaxation that supports fluid, effortless movement. This relaxation response not only reduces muscular tension but also cultivates a sense of ease and well-being in daily activities.

the principles of somatic exercises underscore the holistic nature of movement and well-being, integrating the mind, body, and awareness into a unified approach to movement education.

By understanding these principles and engaging in somatic practices, individuals can unlock greater potential for mobility, reduce pain and tension, and cultivate a deeper connection with themselves.

CHAPTER 2
Exploring Body Awareness

Exploring Body Awareness in the context of somatic exercises for beginners involves delving into the intricacies of how individuals perceive and interact with their bodies. This exploration encompasses various aspects such as body scanning techniques, developing sensory awareness, and recognizing patterns of tension and stress.

Body scanning techniques are fundamental in somatic practices as they facilitate a deep connection between the mind and body. Beginners are often introduced to systematic body scans where they focus their attention on different parts of their body sequentially. This process encourages individuals to notice subtle sensations, tensions, or areas of ease within their bodies.

By systematically scanning through each body part, from head to toe or vice versa, beginners can cultivate a heightened awareness of their physical state, paving the way for a more holistic understanding of their body-mind connection.

Developing sensory awareness is another key concept in somatic exercises for beginners. It involves honing the ability to perceive and interpret sensory information from within the body.

This includes sensations such as touch, temperature, pressure, proprioception (awareness of body position), and interoception (awareness of internal bodily sensations like hunger or heart rate).

Through guided somatic exercises, beginners learn to tune into these sensory cues, fostering a deeper understanding of how their bodies respond to various stimuli. This heightened sensory awareness can lead to improved posture, movement coordination, and overall body alignment.

Recognizing patterns of tension and stress is an essential aspect of body awareness in somatic practices.

Beginners are encouraged to observe and identify habitual patterns of tension or areas of stress within their bodies.

This involves noticing areas that feel tight, restricted, or uncomfortable during movement or at rest.

By acknowledging these patterns, individuals can begin to unravel underlying causes such as posture habits, emotional stressors, or past injuries.

Through somatic exercises focused on releasing tension and promoting relaxation, beginners can gradually transform these patterns, leading to a more balanced and harmonious relationship with their bodies.

Exploring body awareness in somatic exercises for beginners involves introducing techniques such as body scanning, developing sensory awareness, and recognizing patterns of tension and stress.

These concepts form the foundation for a deeper understanding of how the mind and body interconnect, ultimately promoting physical well-being and mindfulness in daily life.

CHAPTER 3
Breathing And Relaxation

Breathing and relaxation techniques play a crucial role in somatic exercises for beginners, offering a gateway to enhancing body awareness, reducing stress, and promoting overall well-being.

Among these techniques, diaphragmatic breathing exercises, progressive relaxation techniques, and mindfulness practices for relaxation stand out as foundational tools for beginners embarking on their somatic journey.

Diaphragmatic breathing, also known as abdominal or deep breathing, forms the basis of many relaxation and mindfulness practices.

It involves engaging the diaphragm, a dome-shaped muscle located beneath the lungs, to draw air deep into thc lungs, allowing for more efficient oxygen exchange and a calming effect on the nervous system. Beginners often start with simple diaphragmatic breathing exercises, such as lying on their back with one hand on the abdomen and the other on the chest, focusing on inhaling deeply through the nose and exhaling slowly through the mouth while feeling the rise and fall of the abdomen.

Progressive relaxation techniques are another fundamental aspect of somatic exercises for beginners. These techniques involve systematically tensing and then relaxing different muscle groups in the body, promoting awareness of muscle tension and release.

Beginners can practice progressive relaxation by starting with their feet and working their way up through the legs, abdomen, chest, arms, and finally, the face, consciously tensing each muscle group for a few seconds before relaxing completely. This process not only helps in physical relaxation but also enhances body-mind connection as individuals become more attuned to their bodily sensations.

Mindfulness practices for relaxation further deepen the somatic experience for beginners. Mindfulness involves non-judgmental awareness of the present moment, including thoughts, feelings, bodily sensations, and the surrounding environment.

In the context of relaxation, mindfulness practices often incorporate focused attention on breathing, body scans to notice areas of tension or discomfort, and gentle movement or stretching with full awareness. Beginners can benefit greatly from mindfulness practices as they learn to cultivate a sense of calm, improve concentration, and develop resilience in dealing with stressors.

Combining these three concepts—diaphragmatic breathing exercises, progressive relaxation techniques, and mindfulness practices for relaxation—creates a comprehensive approach to enhancing relaxation and body awareness in somatic exercises for beginners.

As individuals delve deeper into these practices, they not only experience immediate benefits like reduced stress and increased relaxation but also lay a strong foundation for ongoing somatic exploration and growth.

Somatic exercises for beginners encompass a range of principles and techniques aimed at fostering body awareness, enhancing movement efficiency, and promoting overall well-being. Among these principles, body awareness stands out as a foundational concept that underpins the entire somatic experience. Body awareness involves the conscious perception and understanding of one's body, including its sensations, movements, and posture.

One key aspect of body awareness in somatic exercises for beginners is proprioception, the ability to sense the position, movement, and tension of muscles and joints without relying solely on visual cues.

Proprioception plays a vital role in movement quality, coordination, and injury prevention.

Beginners can enhance proprioceptive awareness through various somatic exercises, such as slow and controlled movements that focus on sensing the position of body parts in space, exploring different ranges of motion, and gradually increasing movement complexity over time.

Another important component of body awareness is kinesthetic awareness, which involves the perception of body movements and their relation to the environment.

Kinesthetic awareness allows beginners to coordinate movements effectively, maintain balance, and adapt to changes in their surroundings. Somatic exercises that emphasize mindful movements, such as tai chi, qigong, or somatic yoga, can help beginners develop kinesthetic awareness by encouraging slow, deliberate movements with attention to alignment, breath, and sensation.

In addition to proprioception and kinesthetic awareness, body awareness in somatic exercises for beginners also encompasses sensory awareness, which involves tuning into bodily sensations like touch, temperature, pressure, and pain.

Developing sensory awareness allows beginners to recognize areas of tension, discomfort, or imbalance in the body, which can guide them in choosing appropriate somatic practices and techniques for relaxation, release, and healing.

Overall, body awareness serves as a cornerstone of somatic exercises for beginners, facilitating a deeper understanding of the body-mind connection and paving the way for increased movement proficiency, relaxation, and holistic well-being.

By cultivating body awareness through proprioceptive, kinesthetic, and sensory practices, beginners can embark on a transformative journey of self-discovery, self-care, and embodied presence.

The concept of adaptability is integral to somatic exercises for beginners, offering a flexible and personalized approach to movement, relaxation, and overall well-being. Adaptability in somatic refers to the ability to modify and adjust exercises, techniques, and practices according to individual needs, abilities, goals, and preferences.

One key aspect of adaptability in somatic exercises for beginners is the ability to tailor movements and exercises to suit different body types, fitness levels, and physical abilities.

Beginners may have varying levels of flexibility, strength, mobility, and coordination, making it essential to offer modifications and variations that allow everyone to participate safely and comfortably. For example, in a somatic yoga class, beginners can be offered options to modify poses based on their flexibility and mobility, such as using props like blocks or straps, adjusting the range of motion, or choosing alternative poses that achieve similar benefits.

Adaptability also extends to accommodating individual preferences and goals within somatic practices. Beginners may have diverse motivations for engaging in somatic exercises, such as stress reduction, pain management, improving posture, enhancing athletic performance, or simply exploring new ways of moving and being in their bodies.

By providing a range of exercises, techniques, and approaches, instructors and practitioners can support beginners in finding what resonates best with their needs and interests, fostering a sense of ownership and empowerment in their somatic journey.

Furthermore, adaptability in somatic exercises for beginners encompasses the ability to integrate feedback and reflection into practice sessions. Beginners benefit from opportunities to reflect on their experiences, receive feedback from instructors or peers, and make adjustments accordingly. This reflective process helps beginners refine their movement patterns, deepen their body awareness, and make meaningful progress toward their goals over time.

In essence, adaptability lies at the heart of somatic exercises for beginners, ensuring inclusivity, customization, and continuous learning and growth. By embracing adaptability as a guiding principle, beginners can approach somatic practices with curiosity, openness, and a willingness to explore and evolve their movement and mindfulness practices in ways that are meaningful and sustainable for them.

CHAPTER 4
Basic Somatic Exercises

Basic somatic exercises form the foundational elements of somatic movement practices, focusing on enhancing body awareness, releasing tension, improving posture, and promoting overall well-being. These exercises target specific areas of the body, such as the neck and shoulders, spinal alignment and mobility, and hip and pelvic floor awareness. Each of these concepts plays a crucial role in cultivating a deeper understanding of somatic movement and its benefits for beginners.

The Neck and Shoulder Release exercises are designed to address common areas of tension and stress that many individuals experience due to modern lifestyle factors such as prolonged sitting, computer work, and emotional stress.

These exercises often involve gentle movements, stretches, and self-massage techniques aimed at releasing tight muscles, improving circulation, and restoring flexibility in the neck and shoulder region. By practicing these exercises regularly, beginners can alleviate discomfort, improve their range of motion, and promote relaxation in these areas.

Spinal alignment and mobility are fundamental aspects of somatic movement, emphasizing the importance of maintaining a balanced and functional spine. Somatic exercises for spinal alignment often focus on gentle movements that encourage the vertebrae to move in their natural range of motion, promoting flexibility, strength, and stability.

These exercises may include spinal twists, arches, curls, and lateral movements that help release tension, improve posture, and enhance overall spinal health. Beginners benefit from these exercises by developing greater awareness of their spinal alignment, reducing back pain, and improving movement efficiency.

Hip and pelvic floor awareness are key components of somatic practices that contribute to core stability, balance, and pelvic health. Somatic exercises targeting the hips and pelvic floor aim to release tension, increase flexibility, and improve coordination in these areas.

These exercises often involve gentle hip rotations, pelvic tilts, and pelvic floor contractions to enhance awareness of these muscle groups and promote better alignment and function.

Beginners can experience improved hip mobility, reduced pelvic discomfort, and enhanced pelvic floor strength through regular practice of these exercises.

basic somatic exercises focusing on the neck and shoulders, spinal alignment, and hip and pelvic floor awareness are essential for beginners to develop a strong foundation in somatic movement. These exercises offer numerous benefits, including tension relief, improved posture, enhanced mobility, and increased body awareness.

By incorporating these exercises into their daily routine, beginners can experience the transformative effects of somatic practices on their physical and mental well-being.

CHAPTER 5
Movement Exploration

Movement exploration in somatic exercises for beginners is a foundational concept that emphasizes the quality of movement over quantity. It involves delving into the nuances of how the body moves, feels and responds to different stimuli.

Central to this concept is the practice of slow and controlled movements, which allow individuals to deepen their awareness of bodily sensations and movements. This approach contrasts with traditional exercise paradigms that often prioritize speed and intensity, focusing instead on mindful engagement with each movement.

One key aspect of movement exploration is the emphasis on joint articulation exercises.

These exercises target specific joints in the body, such as the shoulders, hips, knees, and spine, to improve the range of motion, flexibility, and overall joint health.

By consciously moving each joint through its full range of motion in a controlled manner, participants can enhance their proprioception and kinesthetic awareness, leading to more fluid and coordinated movements.

Integrating fluidity and ease is another fundamental aspect of movement exploration in somatic exercises. Rather than approaching movement as a series of isolated actions, this concept encourages individuals to cultivate a sense of flow and continuity in their movements.

By connecting movements seamlessly and transitioning between different positions with grace and ease, practitioners can experience a sense of harmony and integration within their bodies.

Incorporating slow and controlled movements into somatic exercises allows beginners to develop a deep understanding of their body's capabilities and limitations. This approach promotes mindfulness and body awareness, helping individuals to tune into subtle sensations and feedback from their bodies.

By moving slowly and deliberately, participants can identify areas of tension, stiffness, or imbalance, allowing them to address these issues and work towards greater overall movement proficiency.

Joint articulation exercises play a crucial role in movement exploration by targeting specific areas of the body that are commonly affected by stiffness or limited range of motion. These exercises often involve gentle rotations, circles, and oscillations to mobilize the joints and surrounding tissues.

By regularly practicing joint articulation exercises, beginners can improve joint mobility, reduce stiffness, and enhance their overall movement quality.

Integrating fluidity and ease into somatic exercises encourages participants to move with a sense of flow and naturalness.

This approach emphasizes smooth transitions between movements, avoiding jerky or abrupt actions that can lead to strain or injury.

By focusing on fluid movement patterns, individuals can cultivate a sense of relaxation and ease in their bodies, promoting a more efficient and enjoyable movement experience.

Overall, movement exploration in somatic exercises for beginners offers a holistic approach to movement that prioritizes mindful awareness, joint health, and fluidity of motion.

By incorporating slow and controlled movements, joint articulation exercises, and integrating fluidity and ease, participants can enhance their movement capabilities, reduce tension and discomfort, and develop a deeper connection with their bodies.

This approach can be particularly beneficial for individuals seeking to improve mobility, flexibility, and overall well-being through gentle and mindful movement practices.

CHAPTER 6
Somatics For Stress Reduction

Somatic exercises offer a holistic approach to stress reduction, integrating the mind and body to promote overall well-being. In the realm of somatics, stress relief is not just about temporary relaxation but aims for a deeper transformation in how we perceive and respond to stressors.

This section delves into various concepts related to somatic practices for stress reduction, including stress-relief techniques, calming the nervous system, and the profound impact of somatics on mental and emotional well-being.

Stress-Relief Techniques

Somatic stress-relief techniques encompass a wide range of practices designed to release tension, enhance body awareness, and foster relaxation. These techniques often involve gentle movements, breathing exercises, mindfulness practices, and body scanning. One key aspect of somatic stress relief is the focus on sensing and feeling the body rather than just intellectually understanding stress. By engaging in somatic practices, individuals can develop a heightened awareness of how stress manifests physically and learn to release tension at a deep level.

Breathing techniques play a significant role in somatic stress relief. Practices such as diaphragmatic breathing, where one focuses on deep, slow breaths that engage the diaphragm fully, can help calm the nervous system and reduce stress levels. Mindful breathing, which involves paying attention to the inhales and exhales without judgment, can also be incorporated into somatic exercises to promote relaxation and present-moment awareness.

Movement is another powerful tool in somatic stress relief. Gentle, mindful movements that emphasize fluidity and ease can help release physical tension accumulated from stress. Practices like somatic yoga, tai chi, or simple body-awareness exercises can be effective in promoting relaxation and reducing the impact of stress on the body.

Calming the Nervous System

The nervous system plays a central role in our response to stress. Somatic exercises target the nervous system by promoting a state of relaxation and reducing the activation of the sympathetic nervous system, which is responsible for the body's fight-or-flight response.

Calming the nervous system through somatic practices involves activating the parasympathetic nervous system, often referred to as the "rest and digest" mode.

One approach to calming the nervous system through somatics is through progressive relaxation techniques. These techniques involve consciously tensing and then relaxing different muscle groups, promoting a sense of release and relaxation throughout the body.

By systematically engaging with different parts of the body, individuals can become more attuned to areas of tension and learn to let go of stress-related muscle tightness.

Another way somatics calm the nervous system is by promoting body awareness and proprioception. Proprioception refers to the body's ability to sense its position in space. Somatic exercises that focus on proprioceptive awareness can help individuals become more mindful of their body's responses to stress and learn to regulate these responses more effectively.

Mental and Emotional Well-Being with Somatics

Beyond physical relaxation, somatics also significantly impact mental and emotional well-being. The mind-body connection inherent in somatic practices allows individuals to explore and address the emotional aspects of stress.

By bringing awareness to physical sensations, emotions, and thought patterns, somatics offers a pathway to understanding and transforming stress at a deeper level.

One aspect of somatic mental well-being is the cultivation of mindfulness. Mindfulness practices, integrated into somatic exercises, encourage individuals to observe their thoughts and emotions without judgment, promoting a sense of acceptance and resilience in the face of stressors. This non-reactive awareness can help break habitual patterns of stress reactivity and foster a more adaptive response to challenging situations.

Somatic also promote emotional regulation by providing tools to navigate intense emotions that often accompany stress. Through practices like body scanning, individuals can learn to identify areas of tension associated with specific emotions and work towards releasing these tensions through mindful movement and breathwork.

This process supports emotional resilience and a greater sense of emotional balance.

Somatic exercises offer a multifaceted approach to stress reduction, addressing physical tension, calming the nervous system, and promoting mental and emotional well-being. By integrating somatic practices into daily life, individuals can cultivate a deeper connection with themselves, enhance their ability to manage stress effectively and foster a sense of overall balance and resilience.

CHAPTER 7
Somatics For Pain Management

In the realm of somatic exercises, a profound area of focus lies in pain management, particularly concerning chronic pain. Chronic pain, a multifaceted phenomenon, encompasses persistent discomfort lasting beyond the expected time for healing. Understanding the complexities of chronic pain is paramount for effective management through somatic exercises.

Chronic pain transcends mere physical sensations, delving into the realms of psychology, neurology, and individual experiences. It often defies conventional medical treatments, necessitating a holistic approach that somatic exercises adeptly offer. By addressing not just the symptoms but also the underlying causes and contributing factors, somatics provides a promising avenue for long-term pain relief and improved quality of life.

One of the core principles in somatics for pain management is the recognition of the mind-body connection. This interconnectedness underscores the influence of psychological factors such as stress, anxiety, and trauma on pain perception and tolerance. Somatic exercises, therefore, encompass not just physical movements but also mindfulness practices that promote relaxation, stress reduction, and emotional well-being. By integrating these elements, somatics offers a comprehensive approach to pain management that goes beyond traditional physical therapies.

Gentle exercises play a pivotal role in somatic pain management. Unlike high-impact or strenuous workouts that may exacerbate pain, somatic exercises emphasize gentle, mindful movements aimed at restoring functional movement patterns, reducing muscle tension, and improving body awareness. These exercises often involve slow, controlled movements combined with focused breathing and relaxation techniques.

By engaging in these gentle exercises regularly, individuals can gradually retrain their bodies, alleviate pain, and improve mobility without causing additional strain or discomfort.

Addressing common pain conditions is a central aspect of somatic pain management. Conditions such as lower back pain, neck and shoulder tension, joint pain, and fibromyalgia are prevalent challenges that many individuals face.

Somatic exercises offer tailored approaches to address these specific pain conditions, taking into account individual differences in movement patterns, muscle imbalances, and pain triggers. Through targeted exercises that focus on releasing the tension, improving posture, and enhancing body awareness, somatics empowers individuals to manage their pain more effectively and regain control over their bodies.

Lower back pain, a widespread issue with a significant impact on daily life, is a primary target for somatic pain management strategies. Somatic exercises for lower back pain often include gentle stretches, mobility drills, and awareness-building movements that target the muscles and fascia surrounding the lumbar spine.

By addressing muscular imbalances, improving spinal alignment, and promoting proper movement mechanics, somatics can help alleviate lower back pain and prevent future flare-ups.

Neck and shoulder tension, commonly associated with sedentary lifestyles, poor posture, and stress, is another area where somatic exercises excel. These exercises focus on releasing tension in the neck, shoulders, and upper back through gentle movements that promote relaxation, increase mobility, and improve posture awareness. By incorporating mindful breathing and relaxation techniques, somatic exercises for neck and shoulder tension offer a holistic approach to reducing pain and enhancing overall well-being.

Joint pain, whether due to arthritis, injury, or overuse, can significantly impact mobility and quality of life. Somatic exercises for joint pain target specific joints such as the knees, hips, and shoulders, using gentle movements and range-of-motion exercises to improve joint flexibility, reduce inflammation, and increase functional capacity. By promoting joint health through mindful movement and body awareness, somatics can help individuals manage joint pain and maintain an active lifestyle.

Fibromyalgia, a chronic condition characterized by widespread musculoskeletal pain, fatigue, and sleep disturbances, poses unique challenges for pain management. Somatic exercises for fibromyalgia focus on gentle, low-impact movements that alleviate muscle stiffness, improve circulation, and enhance relaxation. These exercises also incorporate elements of mindfulness and stress reduction to address the psychological aspects of fibromyalgia, such as anxiety and depression. By providing a holistic approach that addresses both physical and emotional aspects of fibromyalgia, somatics offers a comprehensive strategy for managing this complex condition.

Somatic exercises for pain management offer a holistic and integrative approach to addressing chronic pain conditions. By understanding the complexities of chronic pain, incorporating gentle exercises, and targeting common pain conditions, somatics empowers individuals to take control of their pain, improve their quality of life, and promote overall well-being.

CHAPTER 8
Somatic Adaptability

Somatic adaptability refers to the capacity of the body and mind to adjust and respond effectively to changes in movement patterns, environmental demands, and internal states. In the context of somatic exercises for beginners, adaptability plays a crucial role in enhancing flexibility, improving posture, managing stress, and promoting overall well-being.

One of the fundamental principles of somatic adaptability is neuroplasticity, which refers to the brain's ability to reorganize itself by forming new neural connections throughout life. Through consistent practice of somatic exercises, individuals can stimulate neuroplasticity, leading to improved motor control, increased body awareness, and enhanced movement efficiency. This adaptability extends beyond physical movements to encompass mental and emotional resilience, allowing individuals to navigate challenges with greater ease and flexibility.

Somatic exercises for adaptability often focus on mindful movement, breath awareness, and sensory perception. Practices such as the Feldenkrais Method and Hanna Somatics emphasize gentle, exploratory movements that encourage the nervous system to relearn optimal movement patterns. By engaging in these exercises, beginners can gradually release habitual muscular tension, correct imbalances, and improve coordination.

Furthermore, somatic adaptability involves cultivating a mindset of curiosity and experimentation. Beginners are encouraged to approach each exercise with an open mind, noticing subtle sensations and observing how their bodies respond. This process of self-discovery not only enhances adaptability but also fosters a deeper connection between body, mind, and environment.

Somatic adaptability is about embracing change, learning from experience, and continuously evolving toward greater ease and functionality in movement and life.

Modifying Exercises for Individual Needs

When embarking on a journey of somatic exercises, it's essential to recognize that each individual has unique needs, abilities, and limitations. Modifying exercises to suit individual needs is not only practical but also promotes safety, effectiveness, and long-term adherence to the practice.

One of the key aspects of modifying somatic exercises is tailoring them to accommodate physical capabilities and any pre-existing conditions. Beginners may have varying degrees of flexibility, strength, and mobility, requiring adjustments in intensity, range of motion, or duration of exercises. For example, someone with limited mobility in the shoulders may modify arm movements to a comfortable range, focusing on gentle stretching and gradual improvement over time.

Additionally, modifications can be made to address specific goals or areas of focus. For instance, individuals seeking stress relief may benefit from incorporating breathwork and relaxation techniques into their somatic practice. Those aiming to improve posture may emphasize exercises that target the core muscles and promote spinal alignment.

Furthermore, modifications consider the holistic well-being of individuals, taking into account factors such as emotional state, energy levels, and personal preferences. Beginners are encouraged to listen to their bodies, communicate any discomfort or challenges to instructors or guides, and make adjustments as needed to ensure a positive and empowering experience.

Overall, modifying exercises for individual needs is a cornerstone of effective somatic practice, promoting inclusivity, accessibility, and personalized growth for beginners and experienced practitioners alike.

Somatics for Different Fitness Levels

Somatics encompasses a wide range of exercises and practices that can be adapted to suit different fitness levels, from beginners with limited mobility to advanced practitioners seeking greater refinement and depth in their movements. By tailoring somatics to different fitness levels, individuals can experience progressive benefits, improved performance, and a deeper understanding of their bodies.

For beginners, somatic exercises often focus on foundational movements, breath awareness, and gentle stretches. These practices introduce fundamental concepts such as sensory perception, neuromuscular coordination, and relaxation techniques. Beginners may start with simple exercises that emphasize body scanning, proprioception, and mindful movement, gradually building strength, flexibility, and body awareness over time.

Intermediate practitioners in somatics may explore more complex movements, variations, and sequences that challenge coordination, balance, and proprioceptive feedback. These exercises may involve integrating multiple body parts, exploring different planes of movement, and transitioning between static and dynamic positions. Intermediate-level somatics often emphasizes fluidity, precision, and integration of breath with movement, enhancing overall functional fitness and mind-body connection.

Advanced somatic practices are characterized by refined awareness, subtle adjustments, and mastery of intricate movement patterns. Advanced practitioners may delve into advanced techniques such as pandiculation, where they actively contract and release muscles to reset neuromuscular patterns and improve motor control.

These practices require a high level of focus, discipline, and self-regulation, leading to profound shifts in movement efficiency, emotional resilience, and somatic intelligence.

Regardless of fitness level, somatics offers a holistic approach to fitness and well-being, emphasizing quality of movement, mindfulness, and self-care. By embracing somatics at different levels, individuals can discover new depths of physical potential, cultivate resilience, and experience a profound sense of embodiment and vitality.

Incorporating Somatics into Daily Life

The integration of somatics into daily life extends beyond structured exercise sessions to encompass mindful movement, body awareness, and self-care practices that promote well-being and vitality throughout the day.

By weaving somatic principles into everyday activities, individuals can enhance their physical, mental, and emotional resilience, leading to a more balanced and fulfilling lifestyle.

One of the key aspects of incorporating somatics into daily life is cultivating mindfulness in movement. This involves paying attention to body sensations, posture, and breath during routine activities such as walking, sitting, and standing.

By bringing awareness to habitual movement patterns and making subtle adjustments, individuals can reduce muscular tension, improve alignment, and prevent strain or injury.

Breath awareness is another integral component of somatic integration. Practicing mindful breathing techniques throughout the day can help regulate stress levels, promote relaxation, and enhance the oxygenation of tissues.

Simple practices such as diaphragmatic breathing, square breathing, or mindful breath counting can be seamlessly integrated into work, leisure, or rest periods, fostering a sense of calm and presence.

Furthermore, somatics encourages regular movement breaks and micro-practices that counteract the effects of sedentary behavior. Incorporating short movement sequences, stretches, or self-massage techniques into daily routines can improve circulation, alleviate stiffness, and boost energy levels. These micro-practices serve as gentle reminders to prioritize self-care and physical well-being amidst busy schedules.

In addition to physical practices, somatic integration involves nurturing a positive mindset and emotional resilience. Cultivating gratitude, self-compassion, and mindful awareness of thoughts and emotions can enhance overall resilience, mental clarity, and emotional balance. Incorporating moments of reflection, journaling, or meditation into daily life can promote self-discovery, growth, and inner peace.

Overall, incorporating somatics into daily life is about fostering a holistic approach to health and well-being that integrates mindful movement, breath awareness, self-care practices, and emotional resilience. By embracing somatic principles throughout the day, individuals can cultivate a deeper connection with their bodies, enhance vitality, and thrive in all aspects of life.

CHAPTER 9
Mindfulness And Movement

Mindfulness and movement are intertwined concepts that form the core of somatic exercises for beginners. Mindfulness refers to the practice of being present and aware of one's thoughts, feelings, sensations, and surroundings without judgment. Movement, on the other hand, encompasses physical actions and exercises that promote mobility, flexibility, strength, and overall well-being. When combined, mindfulness and movement create a powerful synergy that enhances the mind-body connection and fosters a deeper understanding of oneself.

In somatic exercises for beginners, mindfulness is applied to movement in several ways. First and foremost, beginners are encouraged to cultivate a mindful attitude towards their bodies and movements. This involves paying attention to bodily sensations, exploring range of motion with curiosity, and acknowledging any areas of tension or discomfort without forcing or pushing beyond limits. By practicing mindfulness in movement, beginners develop a heightened sense of body awareness and proprioception, which are essential for safe and effective somatic exercises.

Another aspect of mindfulness in somatic exercises is the focus on breath. Mindful breathing techniques are integrated into movements to promote relaxation, reduce stress, and enhance the mind-body connection. Beginners are guided to synchronize their breath with movement, such as inhaling deeply during expansion or extension and exhaling slowly during contraction or relaxation. This rhythmic breathing pattern not only supports the flow of movement but also calms the nervous system and fosters a sense of calm and centeredness.

Furthermore, mindfulness in somatic exercises extends to the quality of attention and intention brought to each movement. Beginners are encouraged to approach exercises with a non-judgmental attitude, letting go of expectations or self-criticism. Instead, they are invited to embrace a sense of curiosity, playfulness, and openness to new experiences. This mindful approach allows beginners to explore movement patterns, discover areas of tension or restriction, and cultivate a sense of agency and empowerment over their bodies.

Overall, mindfulness and movement are foundational principles in somatic exercises for beginners, shaping the way they interact with their bodies, movements, and inner experiences. By practicing mindfulness in movement, beginners not only improve physical fitness and mobility but also cultivate mental clarity, emotional balance, and self-awareness, leading to holistic well-being and personal growth.

Mindful Eating Practices

Mindful eating is a practice that encourages individuals to slow down, pay attention to their food, and cultivate awareness of hunger, fullness, and eating habits.

In somatic exercises for beginners, mindful eating practices are integrated as part of a holistic approach to well-being, emphasizing the importance of nourishing the body with intention, awareness, and gratitude.

One of the key principles of mindful eating in somatic exercises is tuning into hunger and satiety cues. Beginners are encouraged to listen to their bodies and eat when they are hungry, rather than out of habit, boredom, or emotional reasons. Likewise, they are guided to pause and check in with their fullness level during meals, practicing mindful portion control and avoiding overeating.

Another aspect of mindful eating in somatic exercises is savoring the sensory experience of food. Beginners are invited to engage all their senses while eating, noticing the colors, textures, flavors, and aromas of each bite.

By slowing down and savoring the moment, they develop a deeper appreciation for food and cultivate a more mindful relationship with eating.

Furthermore, mindful eating practices in somatic exercises include recognizing and addressing emotional eating patterns. Beginners learn to differentiate between physical hunger and emotional cravings, using mindfulness techniques to explore the underlying reasons for eating.

By bringing awareness to their emotions and triggers, they can make conscious choices about food that support their overall well-being.

Integrating mindful eating with somatic exercises also involves creating a nourishing environment for meals. Beginners are encouraged to eat mindfully without distractions, such as TV, phones, or computers, allowing them to focus fully on the eating experience.

This mindful approach fosters a sense of mindfulness in daily life and promotes healthier eating habits over time.

Overall, mindful eating practices complement somatic exercises for beginners by promoting a balanced and mindful approach to nourishment, enhancing the mind-body connection, and supporting overall well-being and vitality.

Walking and Moving with Awareness

Walking and moving with awareness are fundamental aspects of somatic exercises for beginners, emphasizing the importance of mindful movement in daily life. Unlike automatic or unconscious movements, walking and moving with awareness involves paying attention to the body's sensations, alignment, and movement patterns, leading to improved posture, mobility, and overall well-being.

In somatic exercises, beginners are introduced to the concept of walking as a mindful practice. They learn to bring awareness to each step, feeling the contact of the feet with the ground, the rhythm of the gait, and the alignment of the body. By walking mindfully, beginners improve proprioception, balance, and coordination, while also reducing stress and promoting relaxation.

Moving with awareness extends beyond walking to encompass all types of movement in daily life. Beginners are encouraged to approach activities such as sitting, standing, reaching, and bending with mindfulness and intention.

This involves tuning into the sensations of the body, noticing any areas of tension or discomfort, and making conscious adjustments to improve posture and movement efficiency.

Furthermore, somatic exercises for beginners include specific movements and exercises designed to enhance body awareness and mindfulness. These may include gentle stretches, joint mobilization exercises, and mindful movement sequences that promote flexibility, strength, and relaxation. By practicing these exercises regularly, beginners develop a greater sense of body awareness, control, and ease of movement in daily activities.

Integrating somatic exercises with walking and moving with awareness also involves cultivating a mindful attitude toward physical activity. Beginners are encouraged to engage in activities that bring joy, relaxation, and a sense of connection with their bodies, rather than focusing solely on performance or fitness goals.

This mindful approach fosters a positive relationship with movement and supports long-term engagement in a healthy and active lifestyle.

Overall, walking and moving with awareness are essential components of somatic exercises for beginners, promoting mindful movement, improved posture, body awareness, and overall well-being in daily life. By incorporating mindfulness into walking and movement, beginners can enhance their physical, mental, and emotional health, leading to a more balanced and fulfilling lifestyle..

Integrating Somatics with Meditation

Integrating somatics with meditation creates a synergistic practice that combines movement, breath, and mindfulness to promote relaxation, self-awareness, and inner peace. In somatic exercises for beginners, integrating somatics with meditation offers a holistic approach to well-being, addressing both the physical and mental aspects of health.

One of the key elements of integrating somatics with meditation is the focus on body awareness and sensations. Beginners are guided to explore the sensations of their bodies during movement and stillness, noticing areas of tension, ease, or discomfort. By bringing awareness to these sensations without judgment, beginners develop a deeper understanding of their bodies and can release physical and emotional tension through mindful movement and breath.

Breath awareness is another fundamental aspect of integrating somatics with meditation. Beginners learn to synchronize their breath with movement, using the breath as a bridge between body and mind.

This rhythmic breathing pattern promotes relaxation, calms the nervous system, and enhances the mind-body connection during somatic exercises and meditation practices.

Furthermore, integrating somatics with meditation involves cultivating a mindful attitude toward thoughts and emotions.

Beginners are encouraged to observe their thoughts and feelings without attachment or reaction, practicing non-judgmental awareness and acceptance. This mindfulness practice supports emotional resilience, stress reduction, and enhanced self-awareness, creating a foundation for personal growth and well-being.

In somatic exercises for beginners, specific somatic movement sequences and meditation techniques are combined to create integrated practices that address various aspects of health and wellness. These practices may include gentle movements to release tension, breath awareness exercises to promote relaxation, and guided meditation to cultivate mindfulness and inner peace.

Overall, integrating somatics with meditation offers beginners a comprehensive approach to well-being, addressing physical, mental, and emotional aspects of health. By combining mindful movement, breath awareness, and meditation practices, beginners can enhance their overall well-being, reduce stress, and cultivate a deeper sense of self-awareness and inner harmony.

CHAPTER 10
Long-Term Success With Somatics

Long-term success with somatic exercises involves more than just learning the movements; it requires a comprehensive approach that addresses sustainability, goal setting, progress tracking, overcoming challenges, and maintaining motivation. Somatic exercises, which focus on enhancing body awareness, movement efficiency, and mind-body connection, can offer profound benefits when practiced consistently over time. This section delves into the strategies and principles that contribute to long-term success with somatics.

Creating Sustainable Somatic Practices

Creating sustainable somatic practices involves establishing routines and habits that support ongoing growth and development. One key aspect is consistency. Regular practice is essential for reprogramming movement patterns and fostering lasting changes in body awareness and control. This consistency extends beyond the duration of individual sessions; it encompasses integrating somatic principles into daily activities and movements.

Another vital element is adaptability. Somatic exercises should be adaptable to various settings and circumstances. This adaptability allows practitioners to continue their practice even when faced with challenges such as limited time or space. For example, simple somatic movements can be incorporated into daily tasks like sitting at a desk or standing in line, promoting continuous awareness and relaxation throughout the day.

Furthermore, sustainability in somatics involves cultivating a mindful approach. Practitioners are encouraged to focus on the quality of movement and the sensations within their bodies rather than rushing through exercises mechanically. This mindful awareness not only enhances the effectiveness of somatic practices but also fosters a deeper connection between the mind and body, promoting overall well-being.

Creating Objectives and Monitoring Results

Setting clear and achievable goals is fundamental to long-term success in somatic exercises. Goals provide direction and motivation, helping practitioners stay committed to their practice. When setting somatic goals, it's essential to consider both short-term objectives, such as improving specific movements or reducing tension in targeted areas, and long-term goals, such as overall posture improvement or enhanced body awareness.

Tracking progress is integral to goal achievement. This can be done through various methods, such as keeping a journal to record sensations, observations, and insights during practice sessions. Tracking progress allows practitioners to identify patterns, monitor improvements, and adjust their approach as needed.

It also serves as a source of motivation, as visible progress reinforces the benefits of consistent somatic practice.

Additionally, incorporating feedback mechanisms can enhance progress tracking. Seeking feedback from qualified somatic instructors or peers can provide valuable insights and guidance for refining techniques and addressing areas of improvement. Feedback loops contribute to a continuous cycle of learning and growth within somatic practices.

Overcoming Challenges and Staying Motivated

Challenges are inevitable in any long-term endeavor, including somatic practices. Common challenges may include time constraints, distractions, fluctuations in motivation, or encountering plateaus in progress.

Overcoming these challenges requires resilience, adaptability, and a proactive mindset.

One effective strategy is to establish a supportive environment. This may involve creating a dedicated practice space that promotes relaxation and focus, minimizing distractions during practice sessions, or enlisting the support of friends or family members who understand the importance of somatic practice and can provide encouragement and accountability.

Moreover, diversifying somatic routines can help prevent monotony and maintain motivation. Exploring new exercises, and variations, or combining somatics with other movement modalities can keep practice sessions engaging and dynamic. Additionally, setting small, achievable milestones can provide a sense of accomplishment and momentum, keeping practitioners motivated on their somatic journey.

Mindfulness techniques can also be invaluable in overcoming challenges and staying motivated.

Practicing mindfulness during somatic exercises, such as focusing on breath awareness or incorporating meditation practices, can enhance concentration, reduce stress, and cultivate a positive mindset towards challenges and setbacks.

Long-term success with somatic exercises is built on sustainable practices, clear goal setting, diligent progress tracking, resilience in overcoming challenges, and maintaining motivation through mindful approaches.

By incorporating these principles into their somatic journey, practitioners can experience lasting benefits in body awareness, movement efficiency, and overall well-being.

Conclusion

Embracing somatic exercises opens a gateway to profound self-awareness and holistic well-being. Through this manual, you've embarked on a transformative journey, unlocking the secrets of your body-mind connection.

As you delve into the principles of somatic exercises and grasp the intricacies of sensory awareness, you're laying a foundation for lasting change. The gentle yet powerful practices of diaphragmatic breathing, progressive relaxation, and mindful movements become your allies in navigating life's challenges with resilience and grace.

By exploring body awareness and releasing patterns of tension, you not only enhance physical mobility but also cultivate a deep sense of calm and balance within. These practices extend beyond mere exercises; they become a way of life, guiding you toward a more mindful existence.

In your quest for stress reduction and pain management, somatics emerge as a beacon of hope. Through gentle movements and mindfulness techniques, you learn to soothe your nervous system, alleviate chronic discomfort, and reclaim joy in everyday moments.

Adaptability becomes your superpower as you tailor somatic exercises to your unique needs and fitness levels. Whether you're a beginner or a seasoned practitioner, integrating somatics into your daily routine becomes second nature, fostering long-term success and well-being.

As you embrace mindfulness in movement, from mindful eating to walking with awareness and integrate somatics with meditation, you discover a harmonious blend of body, mind, and spirit.

This harmonization paves the way for sustainable practices, goal achievement, and unwavering motivation on your wellness journey.

In essence, this manual is not just a guide but a catalyst for transformation—a testament to the power of somatic exercises in nurturing a vibrant, balanced, and fulfilling life. Embrace the journey, embrace yourself, and let somatics be your companion in the beautiful dance of self-discovery and growth.

www.ingramcontent.com/pod-product-compliance
Lightning Source LLC
Chambersburg PA
CBHW050829250726
48653CB00006B/2512